More praise for
365 Daily Affirmations for Creative Weight Management

"This small book offers a large helping of self-acceptance, responsible self-care, and love. Providing food for deeper thought, its pithy messages extend beyond eating and weight management to life and living in general. Yager's approach is a celebration of balance, flexibility, and expanded options."
—Abigail H. Natenshon, author of *When Your Child Has an Eating Disorder*

"Insightful. Gentle in tone, yet rich in meaning, these daily affirmations guide the reader toward healthier eating habits by addressing the 'inner hunger' experienced by us all."
—Reader from Texas

Selected Nonfiction Books by Jan Yager
(a/k/a J.L. (Janet) Barkas)
Friendshifts®: The Power of Friendship and How It Shapes Our Lives
Creative Time Management for the New Millennium
Sleeping Well (with Michael J. Thorpy, M.D.)
Meatless Cooking: Celebrity Style
The Vegetable Passion: A History of the Vegetarian State of Mind
Business Protocol
Effective Business & Nonfiction Writing
Single in America
The Help Book
Victims

Fiction
The Binge
Just Your Everyday People (with Fred Yager)
Untimely Death (with Fred Yager)

Journals
Time to Lose Journal
Personal Journal
Friendship Journal
The Birthday Book
Everything Notebook

365 DAILY AFFIRMATIONS FOR CREATIVE WEIGHT MANAGEMENT

Jan Yager, Ph.D.

HANNACROIX CREEK BOOKS, INC.
Stamford, Connecticut

This book is dedicated to my loving husband, our sons, our parents and siblings, extended family, my friends, and every woman, man, child, or teen who is dealing with a weight challenge or a related eating disorder.

365 Daily Affirmations for Creative Weight Management
by Jan Yager, Ph.D.
Copyright © 2002 by Jan Yager

Published by: Hannacroix Creek Books, Inc.
1127 High Ridge Road, #110
Stamford, CT 06905-1203
http://www.hannacroixcreekbooks.com
E-mail: hannacroix@aol.com

All rights reserved. No part of this book may be reproduced or transmitted in any form or by any means, electronic or mechanical, including photocopying, recording or by any information storage and retrieval system without written permission from the publisher, except for the inclusion of brief quotations in a review.

LCCN: 00-134608

Library of Congress Cataloging-in-Publication Data
   (Provided by Quality Books, Inc.)

Yager, Jan, 1948-
    365 daily affirmations for creative weight management / Jan Yager.
      1st ed.
      p. cm.
      Three hundred sixty-five daily affirmations for creative weight management.
      Includes bibliographical references.
      ISBN: 1889262-57-9 (trade paperback)

    1. Weight loss--Psychological aspects. 2. Food habits--Psychological aspects. 3. Affirmations.
    4. Remotivation therapy. I. Title. II. Title: Three hundred sixty-five daily affirmations for creative weight management

        RM222.2.Y34 2002   613.2'5'019
                                  QBI00-803

Contents

Disclaimer	vi
Author's Note	vii
Affirmations	1
Resources	121
References	123
About the Author	125

DISCLAIMER

The purpose of this book is to provide inspiration and opinions on the topic covered. It is sold with the understanding that neither the publisher nor the author is engaged in rendering medical, nutritional, psychological, or other professional services. Just as every person is unique, so too is everyone's weight loss and maintenance efforts and challenges. Anyone who decides to deal with overeating, to go on a diet, or to implement other weight-reduction, maintenance, weight-gain strategies, such as exercising, should do so under a doctor's care or as part of a recognized, medically-sound weight reduction program in which your participation, progress, and health can be monitored.

Typographical or content mistakes may inadvertently be contained in this book.

The author and the publisher shall have neither liability nor responsibility to any person or entity with regard to any loss or damage caused, or alleged to be caused, directly or indirectly by the opinions or information contained in this book.

You may put a great deal of time and effort into reading this book and it still may not give you the results you wish. Neither this book nor its author or publisher in any way promise weight loss, maintenance, or any other results.

Author's Note

So many who have weight-related issues feel isolated and alone in their struggle. The key reason I wrote these affirmations was to reach out to anyone who has ever had, or has, a weight or body image challenge, or felt alone in these conflicts, to let you know that you are not alone.

Whether you have 10 pounds to lose, or 20 pounds to gain, whether you have successfully lost a lot of weight and are trying to keep it off, or you just need help with food-related issues during a particularly stressful time, these daily affirmations may be beneficial to you.

Of course you could read one affirmation each day, several affirmations during one day, or just one every once in a while. That is up to you. I just hope that these statements help you and that if they do, that you share your favorite pronouncements with your family members or friends. You might also want to try writing your own affirmations, on your computer, using pen and paper, or in a journal dedicated to these issues, as we all collectively work toward the goal of healthy and satisfying eating habits that enhance our lives and the lives of our loved ones.

Jan Yager, Ph.D.
P.O. Box 8038, Stamford, CT 06905-8038
http://www.janyager.com
http://www.janyager.com/writing

1. I love myself, whatever I weigh and whatever my shape.

2. Yesterday can't be undone. But I can make sure that it is the exception, not tomorrow's rule.

3. I cannot change those who upset, annoy, or disappoint me, but I can change how I react to them.

4. I am training myself to keep track of everything I eat. My body certainly does.

5. I realize that weight loss has a double message: weight loss is a good thing but taking away makes me feel bad.

6. I applaud myself for each step I take in controlling my eating.

7. I am trying to be kind to myself; self-love is the only kind of love I have control over

receiving. I can give love to others but I can not guarantee that they are able or willing to receive it or to return it.

8. I may not be responsible for causing my weight problem, but I am responsible for finding a solution to it.

9. I am being kind to others whether or not they are kind to me.

10. I recommit to my weight loss (or gain, if I need to add

pounds) and maintenance program, and long-term success, each and every day.

11. I am selecting a weight loss and management program that is safe, balanced, healthy, supervised by a healthcare or nutritional expert, and suited to my needs, personality, activity level, and lifestyle.

12. The day may seem long when I'm watching what I eat, especially when I first start a weight management program,

and that's okay. I know if I stick with it, it will become second nature. It will get even a tiny bit easier with practice.

13. I applaud myself for taking the first step, "Day One," and I am waking up each day starting afresh with a renewed determination to my creative weight management program.

14. I am following my program and keeping motivated by varying the foods I eat.

15. I forgive myself for being imperfect.

16. I am writing a list of at least seven things I like about myself that have nothing to do with my appearance. I will remember to reread what I have written down, and to dwell on those seven attributes instead of just focusing on how I look.

17. If I am sad, lonely, overwhelmed, disappointed, anxious, depressed, stressed,

frustrated, or angry, I am trying to deal with those feelings in ways other than overeating or misusing food for soothing, rather than nutritional reasons.

18. I like feeling in control more than feeling out of control and I am trying to find a way to be in control if this has been a challenge for me.

19. As the late psychologist Dr. David Leeds used to say, "If you feel the feelings, you'll get

control over them. You'll master them."

20. I am considering what's worked, or failed, for me in the past as information and I am trying again, making sure my current weight loss (weight gain or maintenance) program is safe and under the care of a physician, nutritionist, eating disorder expert, dietician, healthcare, or weight reduction and maintenance professional whose background and advice I trust.

21. I accept that weight issues are complex problems that require daily and long-term effort to solve.

22. Acceptance by others or self-acceptance should be a positive, but since it is possible to get used to criticism and rejection, acceptance can feel strange and foreign. I have to stay with acceptance long enough to make *those* feelings the more comfortable ones.

23. I try to be a good person and I appreciate myself for making that effort.

24. I give myself permission to stop hating myself because my weight or shape is not some ideal that I aspire to, as I reevaluate whether or not that ideal is a realistic one.

25. I am learning how to prepare foods in a healthy and tasty way so I am less likely to binge on junk food out of boredom or poor preparation.

26. Controlling my weight does not mean the food I eat has to be bland, tasteless, or boring.

27. I am learning from the various diets I've been on, and off, in the past, but everyday I start fresh and anew to control and improve my eating habits.

28. I see my weight control efforts not as a diet but as a lifestyle change; I am learning how to creatively manage my weight for long-term benefits.

29. Everything I learn about weight management is a generality. I am unique so I need to carefully consider how any advice, information, or suggestions from any source—medical, popular press including television, radio, newspapers, and magazines, family members, relatives, friends, co-workers, acquaintances, strangers, over the Internet—applies to me.

30. If I was molested or sexually abused, it was not my fault. I am resolved to no longer punish myself, have mixed feelings about my attractiveness, or hate my body because of what was done to me.

31. The scale is a tool for weight control. It provides information about my current weight, as a way of keeping me in reality. The scale is not something to make me feel good or bad about myself.

32. Losing weight is one of the few losses that are positive. Usually losses are negative, like losing a friend, losing money, or losing a fight. By contrast, I am celebrating the positive loss of weight if I am overweight or obese.

33. I did not gain this weight overnight so it will also take time to lose it, and maintain that weight loss. I am therefore taking it a meal at a time.

34. I may not have gotten all the nurturing I needed as a baby, child, or teen but I can now give myself the nurturing I need now that I am no longer a dependent baby.

35. In addition to taking this weight loss and maintenance program one meal at a time, I am also learning to take it one day at a time. I am striving not to dwell on the past or excessively ruminate and worry about the future. I am

trying to learn the joy of staying focused on the "now".

36. Instead of turning to food when I'm angry, instead of swallowing the rage, I am turning toward whomever I have a grievance with, even if it's just in an imaginary discussion or through a letter that I decide not to mail; I am standing up for myself.

37. I am using writing in a journal or in other formats, such as poetry, fiction, and

correspondence to others or even a letter to myself, to work out my feelings and to help me take control of my food.

38. I am looking at the mixed messages I may have gotten from my mother, father, or other family members about food. When I was growing up, how did those confused messages distort how I viewed food? "I'd be there for you but I can't." "I want to eat anything and everything that I like but I don't want to be fat."

39. I am feeling the feelings; that may help me to lose the excess weight and keep it off. But whether or not it impacts on my weight challenge, feeling the feelings is a positive step even if it may be difficult. If feeling the feelings become too overwhelming for me to do on my own, I am seeking out a qualified mental health professional to help me.

40. Instead of overeating, I am writing a list of three reasons

to stop overeating, to lose weight, and to keep it off.

41. I am staying focused on my weight loss and maintenance goals.

42. I am telling myself that it's possible to enjoy the holidays or go on a vacation without overeating.

43. I am reminding myself that the holidays are about more than just food. The holidays are about tradition and

connecting and reconnecting with those I care about.

44. Holidays are tough on those with a weight challenge so I am being kind to myself.

45. I am trying to focus on people and activities other than food.

46. As the late Dr. David Leeds said, "If you shift, those around you may also shift," so I am focusing on my own shifting and see what happens.

47. I see overeating as a symptom and ask myself: "What's eating *me*?"

48. I am terrific.

49. As I get lighter, I may feel lighter inside as well and that may be scary at first, but I am allowing myself to adjust to that change.

50. I am taking control of my food and my life.

51. I care about others, but I am giving myself permission, when appropriate, to also put myself first.

52. I am controlling my own behavior and letting others know what my boundaries and standards are.

53. I am getting more comfortable saying "no" to others, to food, and to situations that are not in my best interest.

54. I am getting more comfortable *hearing* "no."

55. I like myself. (If I do not yet like myself, I am taking steps to improve my self-esteem.)

56. I forgive myself for having harmed anyone in the past, by accident or on purpose, and I am no longer punishing myself for it.

57. I forgive my parents for anything they failed to do,

because I know they tried their best.

58. I am trying my best to be a good parent.

59. I can learn better eating habits and enjoy creative weight management from this time forward.

60. I do not have to have a weight problem for the rest of my life.

61. I do not have to remain obese for the rest of my life.

62. I can become and remain trim, slim, and healthy.

63. Food is not an enemy. It's something I need to consume to survive and, in moderation and if I make healthy choices, it is one of life's pleasures.

64. I can eat desserts in moderation.

65. Drinking water is a blessing, not a punishment.

66. Exercise is a key to feeling good and controlling my weight, not something to dread.

67. I am identifying my binge foods and, if possible, learning to eat those foods in small doses so I take control away from those foods and give the control back to myself.

68. If it is too hard for me to eat the foods I have identified as my binge foods, if possible, I am eliminating those foods from my diet until I have enough control to avoid the pattern that those foods provoke a self-sabotaging binge.

69. I am befriending food.

70. I am taking control of what I am eating.

71. I am careful about snacking.

72. I am trying to think before I put anything into my mouth.

73. I have a problem with food but I am working on it, every day.

74. I have the power to master creative weight management.

75. I am beautiful.

76. I am smart.

77. I am worthy of having my weight in control.

78. I deserve to have one size of clothes that I really like and that reflect my personality.

79. I deserve to like what I see in the mirror and to enjoy my appearance. I am trying to like and accept my shape and myself.

80. I am beautiful from within.

365 Daily Affirmations for Creative Weight Management

81. I am attractive physically whatever number is on the scale.

82. I am keeping better track of how I'm feeling if I find myself wanting to overeat compulsively, or if I start bingeing, and trying to find other ways to self-soothe besides eating, and to deal with those feelings.

83. I am not making fun of others with a weight problem.

365 Daily Affirmations for Creative Weight Management

84. I am not staring at morbidly obese people because I understand their problem; I feel their pain.

85. I am finding other more productive ways to deal with my need to binge, such as drawing, expressing my feelings, reaching out to others, or taking up a new sport or hobby.

86. I am making exercise a positive part of my life.

87. Exercise doesn't have to be a big deal.

88. I say and believe: "I can, I can, I can."

89. I am keeping track of my weight loss progress with regular weigh-ins and, if that is useful to me, and progress photographs.

90. If I wear clothes with an elastic waist, I am buying pants that are my true size, whatever that size is.

91. I believe I can reach my ideal weight, and stay there.

92. I can picture myself thin, in control, fit, and happy with my appearance and weight loss and maintenance success.

93. I am not crash dieting.

94. I did not become overweight or obese overnight. It is taking time to get to my ideal weight; I am patiently putting in that time.

95. I am eating three balanced, healthy meals a day plus healthy, low-calorie snacks.

96. I am thinking of this weight loss program as a welcome lifetime weight management challenge.

97. I am putting time into planning healthy, tasty meals.

98. I am making the time to go shopping so I don't have an empty refrigerator or

cupboards only filled with junk food thereby increasing the likelihood of going off my program.

99. I am proud that I enjoy eating.

100. I am trying to retrain myself to consider the time and effort that I put into preparing food as a pleasant chore rather than a dreaded one.

101. I am allowing myself to go to restaurants and still creatively manage my weight.

102. I am stocking my refrigerator and cupboards with healthy foods that help me through the "munchies."

103. I am not giving up on this weight challenge!

104. I know this is a lifetime commitment to healthy eating and exercise not a sometime concern.

105. If I go off my program, I am not beating myself up with self-blame. I am getting right back on track.

106. I am writing down everything I eat and drink.

107. I am trying my best to stick to the program I'm following and I appreciate my efforts even if I am imperfect.

108. I am not punishing myself because others wrong me or are jealous of me.

109. I am giving to others without needing them to give back to me.

110. If the program I'm following isn't working for me, I am seeking another one that will work, looking for the guidance or care from a qualified doctor or nutritionist's supervision.

111. I am educating myself about food and nutrition.

112. I am staying focused and positive.

113. I am reminding myself of the mental and physical benefits of exercise.

114. I am putting more activity into each and every day.

115. I am spreading the positive energy I now feel about myself, food, exercise, and

living a healthy life, to those I care about—my family and my friends—and to those I meet.

116. I deserve to like the clothes I buy, whatever my size or shape.

117. I am applying the "I will, I will, I will" philosophy to as many aspects of my life as possible, including my weight challenge.

118. I am not seeing this effort as a quick-fix diet. I see this as a

lifetime commitment to healthy, positive, and creative weight management.

119. If I go off my weight control program, I am getting right back on the path.

120. I am not devaluing or overvaluing my aspirations or myself.

121. I see the number on the scale as information rather than something to feel bad or good about.

122. I love myself despite my imperfections.

123. I accept my weight challenge and devote myself to dealing with it in a healthy way.

124. I am setting a good example of eating and exercise for my spouse and children.

125. I am not jealous of people who seem to be able to "eat anything they want."

126. Overeating is one of the most difficult addictions to overcome because I need to eat to live. I need to learn moderation and modification. I cannot eliminate food all together.

127. I do not feel sorry for myself but, if I do, I try to figure out why and channel that feeling into constructive activities and positive thoughts.

128. I accept that watching my weight is a lifetime concern, and that's okay.

129. I know that reaching my weight loss goal will not guarantee personal or professional success, but getting rid of excess weight that is making me overweight or obese will improve my health and probably extend my life.

130. Getting older is inevitable, but adding excess pounds ages me prematurely.

131. Obesity is unhealthy and something I am able to control.

132. Food can't make up for what I didn't get as a child. Compulsive overeating only makes me feel worse about myself.

133. Food is one of life's many pleasures.

134. Portion control is not a penalty; it's a gift.

135. I am finding ways to deal with my anxiety, guilt, fear, regrets, and stress other than overeating.

136. I am aware that there may be new situations related to food, my appearance, and how others react to me that I may have to deal with when I reach my goal weight, and I will deal with them.

137. Most of all, I am giving love to myself.

138. I deserve to like my appearance, whatever my weight, shape, or clothing size.

139. I deserve to like myself, inside and out.

140. I deserve to have a loving family and at least one devoted friend. If I do not have those relationships, I will try to figure out why and do

something constructive about my situation.

141. I deserve to use, not misuse, food.

142. If others are jealous of me, that's their problem, not mine.

143. I know that every day will always be "Day One." This is a lifelong battle and I am either on the winning or the failing side of it.

144. I am going to continue this weight control challenge until I have only one size of clothes that I maintain consistently.

145. I am learning to accept criticism graciously without being self-deprecating or enraged. I am trying to objectively see criticism as "feedback."

146. I am learning to accept compliments graciously.

147. I am learning to deal with unexpected changes and interruptions without getting completely thrown by the situations. But if I need time to adjust to an unexpected event, I am giving myself permission to take as much time as I need to readjust and readapt.

148. I am trying to use my feelings of envy or jealousy to motivate me rather than shut me down.

149. I am kind toward overweight, obese, and overly thin people because I know their pain. I am kind, not hostile or jealous toward anyone who has the figure that I would like to have.

150. I am learning to eat sensibly and achieve my goal weight for myself, not to please anyone else.

151. I am finally learning how to eat sensibly, whatever my age.

152. I know that "creeping obesity" can happen to anyone. Once the extra pounds are there, it's important to do something about taking the pounds off, safely.

153. I don't want to be a yo-yo dieter ever again.

154. I am substituting new, constructive eating patterns and habits for old, destructive ones.

155. I'm patting myself on my back for taking on this weight loss and maintenance challenge.

156. Each and every day I am renewing my commitment to my weight loss and maintenance challenge.

157. I am applauding myself for every pound I lose and keep off.

158. I remember that staying at my goal weight (unless there is a good reason not to, like becoming pregnant) is as crucial as taking off excess weight in the first place.

159. I don't know what's in store for me in all aspects of my life, but I do know that what I eat, and my weight, are within my control.

160. I am applying to my weight challenge what therapist Allen Wheelis wrote in *How People*

Change: "Action which defines a man, describes his character, is action which has been repeated over and over and so has come in time to be a coherent and relatively independent mode of behavior."

161. The sheer act of doing the right thing over and over again helps increase the likelihood that those changes will become permanent.

162. I'm applying the maxim, "fast off, fast on" to my weight challenge, taking my time to permanently lose, and keep off, the excess weight.

163. Instead of a "crash diet," I am taking my time to lose the weight the right way, to learn good eating habits, to include exercise in my activities, and to keep off those unwanted pounds.

164. Bingeing enables me to reject the food, rather than be

rejected by it, but it is an unhealthy way to deal with my feelings.

165. I am learning to be comfortable with acceptance.

166. I'm trying to learn more about binge eating, so I can overcome it if that is a habit I have fallen into. As Geneen Roth wrote in *Breaking Free from Compulsive Eating:* "Bingeing is a symptom. Once it happens it becomes a problem in itself, but it is

foremost a symptom—a symptom that decisions, feelings, and attitudes about yourself, your relationships, and food that preceded the onset of the binge are not serving you."

167. I am writing down what makes me angry as well as why.

168. I remind myself that obesity is the second leading cause of death; I am doing something about my obesity because I

deserve to live a long and healthy life.

169. I know that an estimated 300,000 Americans die each year directly because of obesity, and that this is an international problem as well, and I want to do what I can to avoid becoming one of them.

170. Although obesity is a national and international problem, I cannot change the world. I can only do my part to deal with my own excess

weight and to set a positive example for my family and friends.

171. I know that the definition of obesity is being 20% above the recommended weight for my height. If I fit into that definition, I will heed the warnings of the documented, increased health risks related to obesity.

172. Rage causes me to overeat, but I am finding

healthier, non-food ways to cope with that feeling.

173. Anger causes me to overeat, but I am finding better non-food ways to deal with that feeling.

174. Frustration makes me want to overeat, but I am dealing with that feeling in a different way than overeating.

175. Joy makes me want to overeat, but I am learning to

feel that feeling without overeating.

176. Panic makes me overeat, but I am finding other non-food ways to deal with panic.

177. Sadness makes me want to overeat, but I am finding another way to cope with sadness.

178. I am learning to enjoy the process of eating: picking the right foods, preparing meals, selecting healthy snacks.

179. Instead of overeating, I am going for a walk.

180. Instead of overeating, I am drawing, using a pencil, charcoal, pen and ink, or colored pencils.

181. Instead of overeating, I am calling a friend.

182. Instead of overeating, I am visiting a friend.

183. Instead of overeating, I am calling a neighbor to say hello.

184. Instead of overeating, I am inviting a neighbor I feel comfortable with over for coffee, tea, or other soft or diet drinks, to take a walk together, to meet at a nearby coffee shop or diner, to go to the movies, or to go to the library.

185. Instead of overeating, I am digging or planting in my garden.

186. Instead of overeating, I am having fun with clay, creating something with my hands.

187. Instead of overeating, I am jumping rope.

188. Instead of overeating, I am working out.

189. Instead of overeating, I am writing a letter, or sending an e-mail, to an old friend.

190. Instead of overeating, I am going on the Internet and

finding a chat room in which I want to participate.

191. Instead of overeating, I am writing a poem.

192. Instead of overeating, I am reading a poem.

193. Instead of overeating, I am finding and rereading old poems I wrote or that I enjoy rereading.

194. Instead of overeating, I am organizing files or cleaning out my "dump" drawer.

195. Instead of overeating, I am going on a bike ride.

196. Instead of overeating, I am going shopping, keeping my budget in mind.

197. Instead of overeating, I am cleaning something I have been meaning to clean—the stove, the bathtub, the kitchen

floor, the hall closet, the basement, or the garage.

198. Instead of overeating, I am rearranging a closet.

199. Instead of overeating, I am asking someone to go for a run, swim, or walk with me.

200. Instead of overeating, I am petting my cat or my dog.

201. Instead of overeating, I am hugging my spouse.

202. Instead of overeating, I am paying attention to my child.

203. Instead of overeating, I am getting a back rub.

204. Instead of overeating, I am giving someone I love a back rub.

205. Instead of overeating, I am taking a hot bubble bath.

206. Instead of overeating, I am going bowling.

207. Instead of overeating, I am taking up a new sport.

208. Instead of overeating, I am reading a short story.

209. Instead of overeating, I am updating my list of birthdays.

210. Instead of overeating, I am doing volunteer work.

211. Instead of overeating, I am tutoring at the local school.

212. Instead of overeating, I am cleaning out the attic or my bedroom clothes closet.

213. Instead of overeating, I am going to a museum.

214. Instead of overeating, I am going to a pet store to look at the fish or the cats and dogs.

215. Instead of overeating, I am going to a concert.

216. Instead of overeating, I am rearranging the books in my bookcases.

217. Instead of overeating, I am becoming part of a local theatrical group.

218. Instead of overeating, I am going to a meeting with those who share my problem.

219. Instead of overeating, I am joining a community chorus.

365 Daily Affirmations for Creative Weight Management

220. Instead of overeating, I am showing and telling my children that I love them.

221. Instead of overeating, I am joining a health club and actually going there to work out, swim, take a class, or just walk on the treadmill while I read or watch TV, if one is nearby.

222. Instead of overeating, I am going to the mall or going window-shopping.

223. Instead of overeating, I am going to the library.

224. Instead of overeating, I am volunteering at the library.

225. Instead of overeating, I am going to a bookstore, to browse through the books, buy a book or magazine, get a cup of coffee, or attend an event sponsored by the bookstore.

226. Instead of overeating, I am baby-sitting for a neighbor or relative who needs a break.

227. Instead of overeating, I am relaxing for five minutes.

228. Instead of overeating, I am meditating.

229. Instead of overeating, I am washing my hair.

230. Instead of overeating, I am brushing my hair.

231. Instead of overeating, I am brushing my teeth, using floss, or a water pic.

232. Instead of overeating, I am picking out a new recipe, buying the ingredients I need, and trying it out.

233. Instead of overeating, I am meeting a friend for coffee.

234. Instead of overeating, I am making a list of my friends and contacting each and every one in some way—by phone, writing a letter, getting together for a visit, or by e-mail.

235. Instead of overeating, I am going through old magazines or books and deciding which ones to read, donate, or recycle.

236. Instead of overeating, I am planning a block party, a birthday party, or a get together for another reason to celebrate.

237. Instead of overeating, I am going to a movie or show.

238. Instead of overeating, I am writing about how I'm feeling, or drawing a picture that describes my emotions.

239. Instead of overeating, I am starting a journal or a diary to chronicle my eating habits and my efforts to deal with my weight challenge.

240. Instead of overeating, I am seeking out a trained professional or a self-help group that helps people with my problem.

241. Instead of overeating, I am putting together stuff for a tag or garage sale or to donate to a charity.

242. Instead of overeating, I am cleaning out the attic.

243. Instead of overeating, I am taking photographs of how I look right now.

244. Instead of overeating, I am organizing the family photograph albums.

245. Instead of overeating, I am going to a lecture on nutrition or reading about healthy eating habits in books, magazines, or on the Internet at sites that I trust.

246. Instead of overeating, I am visiting the aquarium or the zoo.

247. Instead of overeating, I am planning a vacation.

248. Instead of overeating, I am volunteering in a local literacy program.

249. Instead of overeating, I am going on a one-day trip to another town or city.

250. Instead of overeating, I am reading through a magazine or today's newspaper.

251. Instead of overeating, I am rereading old newsletters or newspapers I never get to read through.

252. Instead of overeating, I am writing to my nieces or nephews.

253. Instead of overeating, I am calling my parents and telling them I've been thinking about them. (If my parent or parents are deceased, I am writing a letter, or an essay, to express my feelings about them.)

254. Instead of overeating, I am polishing the furniture.

255. Instead of overeating, I am making a list of foods for today or tomorrow's meals.

256. Instead of overeating, I am planning an "upgrade day" for my computer equipment, or reading over the manuals for the computer or related software that I may not have consulted before.

257. I am taking a cooking course if I need to improve my culinary skills.

258. I am catching myself if I am having a negative thought, and trying to turn it around into a positive one.

259. If I'm having a bad day, I'll remind myself that everyone has bad days, and that I can get through it without compulsively overeating.

260. I am patiently working on eliminating my impatience.

261. I am working on my low tolerance for frustration.

262. I am reaching out to others who share this problem so we can help each other.

263. I am convincing myself that achieving my goal weight, and staying there, is possible. Whether it is easy, or hard, for me to achieve, and maintain, my goal weight, I am committed to that goal.

264. I am making plans for how I will handle situations facing me that present food-related

challenges, such as a family vacation, eating out, attending business breakfasts, lunches, or dinners, parties, or special occasions.

265. I am learning to say "no thank you" without feeling guilty that I'm insulting someone's feelings, especially in food-related situations.

266. I like myself in a bathing suit no matter what I weigh. (But if I do not feel comfortable wearing a bathing suit, I do not

have to explain my decision to anyone else.)

267. I am smiling when I walk by a mirror, whatever I weigh.

268. I am buying a new outfit whatever my current weight, and not "waiting" to start enjoying shopping for clothes.

269. I know that I may plateau on my weight loss from time to time, but I will try not to get discouraged. It is the overall

picture that I'm concerned about.

270. I am trying hard to resist overeating compulsively.

271. I am very carefully considering any claims about "fast" or "easy" solutions to this weight challenge.

272. I will share my success story with others with this problem so they know there is hope.

273. I remember that it is my personality, whether or not I'm a good person, and what I am accomplishing with my life that really counts.

274. I know that losing weight, and keeping it off, may be one of the most difficult challenges I face, but I am approaching this challenge with renewed commitment and optimism.

275. I know there are no easy answers to this weight challenge.

276. I carefully read the labels and the ingredients of all the foods I plan to buy.

277. It is not necessary to suffer to become the weight I want to be.

278. If I need to talk with a professional about the reasons behind my overeating, I am seeking out a therapist without shame or embarrassment.

279. I know there is no one plan or program that will work for everyone.

280. Becoming the weight my body should be is just one way of being kind and loving to myself.

281. I can make it through this day without compulsively overeating.

282. I can make it through this weekend without sabotaging

my weight management efforts.

283. I am not punishing myself for going off my program, but I will get right back on.

284. I know this problem is not a male or female issue or problem.

285. I am more aware of the messages about food that I am passing on to my children.

286. I am making an effort to have reunions and activities exclusive of food.

287. I am creating a list of at least three things about myself that I would like to change that have nothing to do with appearance.

288. I am writing a list of three people I've lost contact with that I'd like to reconnect with (and, if I think it is in my best interest, then somehow will

make the time to reconnect with them).

289. I am writing a list of at least three things about my childhood that were pleasant and memorable. I will try dwelling on those pleasant thoughts if I have been prone to dwelling on the negative aspects of my childhood.

290. I am catching myself every time I say, "What if" about my past. Instead, I embrace my

past but work on changing the present and the future.

291. I am looking for answers within myself, whenever possible.

292. I am embracing a proactive and positive attitude.

293. It's so important, no matter what my weight, that I do not avoid social situations. That way I can avoid the "before" and "after" mentality of thinking life "begins" after I

lose weight. Life is life, and I'm entitled to fully partake in it, whether I'm overweight, obese, a healthy, ideal weight, or thin.

294. When I'm tired, hungry, or frustrated, I have to be especially careful to avoid overeating or turning to food to deal with my problems or needs.

295. I remind myself that creative weight management is all about changing patterns, and

habits. It's about creating different scripts when it comes to food, exercise, body image, self-esteem, and eating.

296. My pantry is easier to stock than my psyche or mind. But I can try to stock my mind or psyche with self-affirming, positive thoughts.

297. I'm trying to take better care of me.

298. I must be doing something right. I need to dwell on what I

am doing right and use that positive reinforcement to work on whatever I want to change or improve.

299. I'm not afraid of being the subject of jealousy, of being perceived as someone without a weight problem, instead of being the one who feels jealous.

300. Life is exciting and I am trying to embrace its wonder rather than fear for tomorrow!

301. Even if I didn't or don't get from others what I needed or need, I can now give it to myself.

302. Instead of looking for love from the inside of the refrigerator, I'm going to love *myself* from the inside.

303. Insight is power and I am working on gaining insight into why I overeat as well as how to overcome my weight challenge and overeating habits.

304. I am ultimately responsible for changing myself. Even a therapist is just a catalyst, or facilitator, for me so I can change myself.

305. I rejoice in the self-control I'm gaining.

306. I'm more willing to direct my anger at the source of that anger by expressing it, appropriately, rather than by eating fattening food that only makes me angry with myself.

But if, especially in business situations, it is wiser to avoid expressing my anger, I will accept that and not swallow the anger along with unnecessary, fattening foods eaten out of rage rather than hunger. I am discovering non-food, advantageous ways to deal with my anger.

307. I need to continue standing up to food each and every day.

308. I am staying focused on my creative weight management goals. It is by making these goals a constant priority that I have a greater probability of achieving, and maintaining, my goals.

309. The self-fulfilling prophecy concept in sociology applies to my weight issues: if I now see myself as someone who is able to control my weight, I am more likely to be able to fulfill that prophecy: I have to believe that I *will* be that way.

310. I am not hiding, no matter what my weight.

311. I am standing tall and walking tall, no matter what my weight.

312. I am patting myself on my back for what I have *already* achieved.

313. Dream it and it can become true.

314. I want to feel healthy and good; I want to look fit and trim.

315. Food, in moderation, is fuel and is pleasurable.

316. Overeating can become an addiction and food, in excess, can become harmful or dangerous. I am dealing with these challenges.

317. I am grateful that I am a nice person.

318. I am grateful that I have a loving family.

319. I am grateful that I have a roof over my head.

320. I am grateful that I am facing my weight challenge and doing something about it.

321. Life doesn't start after I've lost the weight. Life is now. Life is every day.

322. I am lucky to be alive and healthy.

323. I am lucky to be taking on this weight challenge.

324. If I "cheat" or have a "bad day" with food, I'm not beating up on myself. I'm human. I am getting back into control.

325. I am learning to be kind to myself.

326. I am striving to be consistently kind to my family members.

327. I am trying to be kind to those I work for and to my customers, clients, co-workers, or employees.

328. It is so powerful when someone you love really hears you, and feels your pain, and feels your joy. I am trying to be like that with everyone I know and meet.

329. I am working at giving the gift of listening to those I love: to really hear them, to feel their pain, to feel their joy.

330. I am watching out for when I am grabbing food when I'm distressed, bored, or tired.

331. I am attempting to exercise regularly.

332. If possible, I am not skipping meals.

333. I feel so blessed that I am giving myself this renewal by approaching food differently than ever before.

334. I am keeping track of how I'm feeling if I find myself wanting to overeat compulsively, or if I start bingeing. I am finding other ways to deal with those feelings besides turning to food.

335. I am following a weight program that is safe, balanced, and suited to my needs.

336. I am continuing to remind myself, "yes, yes, yes," and

that I can apply the strong will I show in other areas of my life to my creative weight management challenges.

337. I am continuing to find the courage to get on the scale and face the reality of what I weigh.

338. As I lose weight and approach my goal weight, I need to remind myself that reaching my goal weight will not guarantee personal or

professional success or happiness.

339. I am striving to feel compassion toward those who have wronged me.

340. I *can* handle anxiety without turning to food. I *can* handle frustration without turning to food.

341. Those who successfully deal with the problem of obesity need to spread the message to those still

suffering: that change is possible; that there is hope for a healthier, better way of eating and living.

342. I am freeing myself from the shackles of shame, self-hate, and a distorted body image.

343. I look sensational, whatever my size or weight.

344. It is human nature to be pulled back toward what I've lost, but I am resisting that pull

and maintaining my weight loss as a positive change in my life.

345. I applaud myself for my self-determination and pride.

346. I believe in myself.

347. I believe I can successfully manage my weight.

348. I am making healthy, positive decisions about what I am eating today.

349. I am exercising because it is fun and good for me.

350. The future excites me but I'm not living for it.

351. I am grounded in the present; I am not living in the past.

352. I feel calm and if I don't feel calm this minute, I remember when I have felt calm and I am trying to recreate that feeling.

353. I feel peaceful or I am exploring techniques to help me to find inner peace.

354. Some of the things I'm doing I've known before, I've heard before, but I didn't do these things until now. I wasn't ready, until now. Now I'm ready to hear what I need to hear and to do what I need to do.

355. I have to do what I know works for me.

356. Bingeing, unmanaged, turns my life into one long battle with food. I do not want to battle food anymore. I want to be in control of my food and not allow food to control me.

357. I am watching and listening to what triggers my weight challenges.

358. If I work at whatever weight management program I am on, the scale will take care of itself and reflect those efforts.

359. Today I am approaching food with love and excitement, not addiction, anger, or compulsiveness.

360. I can gain control over my weight problem. It's a question of redirecting my focus, then changing my thinking and my actions.

361. I can't change the past, but now I can look forward to the rest of my life being filled with a friendship with food—not a war.

362. Losing weight can bring up uncomfortable feelings. I will stick with those feelings, and work them through in non-food ways, on my own or, if I need help, by seeking out a qualified therapist.

363. I may always have to weigh and measure what I eat, and that's okay. I can creatively manage my weight, thereby choosing to be on the winning side of this weight challenge.

364. I want to set an example for my family by developing a healthy relationship with food. I am their teacher. I am their role model. I do not want to pass on to the next generation the negative attitudes toward food and the habits I've developed that have caused me so much pain during my lifetime.

365. I decide how food fits into my life and whether food is a pleasure and a source of health, nourishment, taste,

and joy rather than a natural function that receives a disproportionate amount of my attention and energy.

Each day, in big and small ways, I have a chance to make sound choices about what I eat, when, and why.

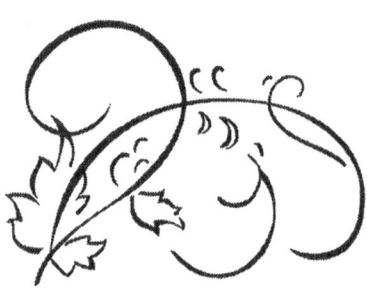

Sources of Information

*Here are selected resources for further information or referrals weight-related concerns:

Academy for Eating Disorders
www.acadeat.org

Eating Disorder Referral and Information Center
http://www.edreferral.com

www.gurze.com (Publisher and bookstore of books related to eating disorders)

International Association of Eating Disorders Professionals
www.iaedp.com

www.nal.usda.gov/fnic/Fpyr/pyramid.html (how to access the United States Department of Agriculture's Food Guide Pyramid)

National Association of Anorexia Nervosa and Associated Disorders
www.anad.org

---

*Please note: Listing of an association, organization, or government agency does not imply an endorsement by the author or publisher. Since a phone number, address, and website may change at any time, and organizations or associations may change name or go out of existence at any time, the accuracy of a listing may not be assured. The author or publisher are not held responsible for any inconvenience that may be caused by an inaccurate or out-of-date listing.

NAAFA (National Association to Advance Fat Acceptance, Inc.)
www.naafa.org

OA (Overeaters Anonymous)
www.overeatersanonymous.org

Weight-Control Information Network
NIH/National Institute of Diabetes and Digestive and Kidney Diseases (NIDDK)
www.niddk.nih.gov/health/nutrit/pubs/binge.htm
(Binge Eating Disorder information)
www.nal.usda.gov/fnic/Fpyr/pyramid.html
(U.S. Dept. of Agriculture's Food Guide Pyramid)

www.weightwatchers.com
Information as well as locations, nationally and internationally, of Weight Watchers® programs closest to where you live.

WINS (We Insist on Natural Shape)
www.winsnews.org

http://www.janyager.com/writing/the_binge.htm
Internet URL of listing of associations and information sources, including web sites and books, created by Jan Yager as an extension of her novel *The Binge*. (See listing below under References.)

Selected References

Brody, Jane E. "Just How Perilous Can 25 Extra Pounds Be?" *The New York Times*, September 20, 1995, page C11.

Chernin, Kim. *The Hungry Self.* New York: HarperPerennial, 1985.

_____. *The Obsession: Reflections on the Tyranny of Slenderness*. New York: Harper & Row, 1982.

Cohen, Mary Anne. *French Toast for Breakfast*. Carlsbad, CA: Gurze Books, 1995.

Davis, Laura. *The Courage to Heal Workbook: For Women and Men Survivors of Child Sexual Abuse*. New York: Harper & Row, 1990.

Gubin, Karin J. with Richard K. Thomas. *Healing the Hungry Heart: The Link between Eating Disorders and Sexual Abuse*. Memphis,TN: MSRG Publications, 1994.

Hollis, Judi. *Fat and Furious: Women and Food Obsession*. New York: Ballantine Books, 1994.

Kallen, David J. and Marvin B. Sussman, editors. *Obesity and the Family*. New York: The Haworth Press, 1984.

Kano, Susan. *Making Peace With Food: Freeing Yourself from the Diet/Weight Obssession.*. Revised edition. New York: Harper & Row, Publishers, 1989.

Maine, Margo. *Father Hunger: Fathers, Daughters & Food.* Carlsbad, CA: Gurze Books, 1991.

Natenshon, Abigail H. *When Your Child Has an Eating Disorder: A Step-By-Step Workbook for Parents and Other Caregivers.* San Francisco, CA: Jossey-Bass, 1999.

Tec, Leon. *The Fear of Success.* New York: New American Library, 1976.

Yager, Jan. *The Binge.* Stamford, CT: Hannacroix Creek Books, Inc., 2002.

_____. *Time to Lose Journal.* Stamford, CT: Hannacroix Creek Books, Inc., 2000.

Wilbert, Jeffrey R. and Norean K. Wilbert. *Fattitudes®: Beat Self-Defeat and Win Your War With Weight.* New York: St. Martins Press, 2001.

Winter, Arthur and Ruth Winter. *Smart Food: Diet and Nutrition for Maximum Brain Power.* New York: St. Martin's Griffin, 1999.

ABOUT THE AUTHOR

JAN YAGER (www.janyager.com) has a doctorate in sociology (City University of New York, 1983), where she was a National Science Foundation predoctoral fellow in medical sociology. She also has an MA in criminal justice and did a year of graduate work in psychiatric art therapy.

Dr. Jan Yager, a member of the National Association of Science Writers and the Academy for Eating Disorders, is the author of numerous nonfiction books including *The Help Book, Victims,* and *Friendshifts®: The Power of Friendship and How It Shapes Our Lives* which led to interviews on The Today Show, The Oprah Winfrey Show, The View, NPR, as well as in *The Wall Street Journal* and *Time.*

Author of *Creative Time Management for the New Millennium,* and a consultant on time mangement, Jan Yager has applied her expertise in time management to the weight management challenge. She puts forth that unique approach in her audio book *Creative Weight Management: An Audio Book* (a book is forthcoming) as well as the innovative weight management journal, *Time to Lose Journal*.

Her published fiction includes the novel *The Binge*, about a successful woman's determination to overcome her eating disorder, and two suspense novels co-authored with her husband Fred Yager: *Untimely Death* and *Just Your Everyday People.*

www.ingramcontent.com/pod-product-compliance
Lightning Source LLC
LaVergne TN
LVHW011423080426
835512LV00005B/238